To Find The Most Common Organisms Involved In Diabetic Foot Infection And Their Sensitivity To Antimicrobial Agents For The Prevention Of Sepsis/Amputation By The Administration Of Empirical Treatment.

Submitted by:

BATCH NO. 08

4th year M.B.B.S

Supervisor: Asst PROF. DR ROMANA Ayub

Department of Community Medicine

Project Director: Syed Shahmeer Raza

Department of Community Medicine

KHYBER MEDICAL COLLEGE, PESHAWAR

SESSION 2014-2015

SYED SHAHMEER RAZA

KHYBER MEDICAL COLLEGE, PESHAWAR.

PROJECT TITLE: To Find The Most Common Organisms Involved In Diabetic Foot Infection And Their Sensitivity To Antimicrobial Agents For The Prevention Of Sepsis/Amputation By The Administration Of Empirical Treatment.

PROJECT SUPERVISOR: Dr. Romana Ayub.

PROJECT DIRECTOR: Syed Shahmeer Raza

PROJECT ASSISTANT DIRECTORS: Rabia Zeb khan.

Faisal Ahmad.

Mahnoor Tariq Khan.

PROJECT FINANCE DIRECTOR: Nayab Kareem.

Asfandiar S.H.Kakakhel

PROJECT IT DIRECTOR: Reesha Khan Khattak.

ROLL NO

MEMBER

73

SYED SHAHMEER RAZA

190

NAYAB KAREEM

285

ARZOO SARDAR

213

TANZEEL UR REHMAN

238

MAHNOOR TARIQ KHAN

219

SAHAR GUL

286

FATIMA AGHA

234

RABIA ZEB KHAN

144

JALWA MAHMOOD

198

ADIL JADOON

58

FAISAL AHMAD

224

ASFANDIAR SHAHRUKH HIJAZ KAKAKHEL

66

REESHA KHAN KHATTAK

BATCH MEMBERS

ACKNOWLEDGMENTS

We are grateful to ALLAH for giving us the strength to complete the research, without HIS will nothing would have been possible. Special thanks to our supervisor Dr. Romana Inam for her guidance. The cooperation of fellows and teachers is indeed appreciated. We are also thankful to all respondents who spared their precious time for filling out questionnaires of our survey. Last but not the least; we would like to thank our parents for their assistance and moral support.

I, Syed Shahmeer Raza, as the batch director would like to extend my gratitude to my dearest friends Daniyal Nadeem and Amer Kamal Hussain for their help in data collection and analysis.

ABSTRACT

A **diabetic foot** is the one that exhibits any pathology that results directly from diabetes mellitus or any long term complication of diabetes mellitus. Presence of several characteristic diabetic foot pathologies is called diabetic foot syndrome.

The organism responsible for a Diabetic foot is clostridium species in the west [1], hence, we need to know the most common organism involved in DF in our setup. Our research project sheds light on the prevalence of most common organism responsible for diabetic infection and to find out their sensitivity to antimicrobial agents to prevent amputation and sepsis by the administration of empirical treatment. The objective of this study was to analyze the bacterial isolates of all patients admitted to **LADY READING HOSPITAL, KHYBER TEACHING HOSPITAL** and **HAYATABAD MEDICAL COMPLEX,** presented with diabetic foot infection in *Wagner grade 2-5.*

Our study design was prospective, **E.Coli** being the subset that mainly represents the bacterial population, isolated, upon culture. We started by formulating a questionnaire that was circulated among the designated groups of people, to check for organism responsible. According to our findings a large number of people presenting with **Diabetic Foot** showed the following results: A **total** of 100 {62 **aerobes** (62%) and 38 **others** (fungal or **anaerobes**) (38%)} were isolated. This research work would hopefully give us deeper insights into further understanding, prevention and treatment of this disorder.

CONTENTS

LIST OF TABLES

LIST OF GRAPHS

39

6

STAPH AUREUS

39

7

MRSA

40

8

MRSA

40

9

MRSA

41

10

PSEUDOMONAS

42

11

PSEUDOMONAS

42

12

PSEUDOMONAS

43

13

LIST OF PIE CHARTS

CHAPTER 1
INTRODUCTION

- The **diabetic foot** that exhibits any pathology that results directly from diabetes mellitus or any long term complication of diabetes mellitus. [2]

- Presence of several characteristic diabetic foot pathologies is called diabetic foot syndrome.

-

- The most serious foot **complications in diabetes** are:

- *Ulceration* (research estimates that the **lifetime incidence** of foot ulcers with in the diabetic community is around **15-25%**) *"Diabetic foot ulcers (DFU) are estimated to effect 15% of all individuals with diabetes during their lifetime and precede almost 85% of all foot amputations.* [3, 4, 5 & 6]

- *Neuropathic* osteoarthropathy.

These are the significant risk factors for lower extremity amputation.

Administration of antimicrobial agents, to which they are sensitive to, is very important part of the management of these patients.

"Of all methods proposed to prevent diabetic foot ulcers, only foot temperature-guided avoidance therapy was found beneficial in RCTs" according to a meta-analysis". [7]

*"Culture is not necessary for initial infection, because early infection is usually due to **<u>Staphylococcus aureus</u>** and/or **<u>streptococci</u>** which can be handled by first choice of 625mg AUGMENTIN 3 times daily for 5 to 7 days".* [8]

Diabetic foot ulcer is a major **<u>complication of diabetes Mellitus</u>**, and probably the major component of the **<u>diabetic foot</u>**. It occurs in 15% of all patients with diabetes and precedes 84% of All diabetes-related lower-leg <u>amputations</u> [9]

The major increase in mortality among diabetic patients observed over the past 20 years is considered to be due to the development of macro and micro vascular complications, including failure of the **wound healing** process. Wound healing is an innate mechanism of action that works reliably most of the time. A key feature of wound healing is stepwise repair of lost **<u>extracellular matrix</u>** (ECM) that forms the largest component of the dermal skin layer. [10]

Controlled and accurate rebuilding is essential to avoid under- or over-healing that may lead to various abnormalities. But in some cases, certain disorders or physiological insult disturbs the wound healing process. **<u>Diabetes mellitus</u>** is one such metabolic disorder that impedes the normal steps of the wound healing process. Many histopathological studies show a prolonged inflammatory phase in diabetic wounds, which cause a delay in the formation of mature **<u>granulation tissue</u>** and a parallel reduction in **<u>wound tensile strength</u>**. [11]

Non-healing chronic diabetic ulcers are often treated with extracellular matrix replacement therapy.

So far, it is a common trend in diabetic foot care domain to use advanced moist wound therapy, bio-engineered tissue or skin substitute, growth factors and negative pressure wound therapy. [12]

No therapy is completely perfect as each type suffers from its own disadvantages. Moist wound therapy is known to promote fibroblast and keratinocyte proliferation and migration, collagen synthesis, early angiogenesis and wound contraction.

At present, there are various categories of moist dressings available such as adhesive backing film, silicone coated foam, hydro gels, hydrocolloids etc.

Unfortunately, all moist dressings cause fluid retention; most of them require secondary dressing and hence are not the best choice for exudative wounds. [13]

To address the physiological deficiencies underlying diabetic ulcer, various tissue engineering technologies have come up with cellular as well as acellular skin replacement products. New therapies in development are also promising, such as platelet rich fibrin wound patch therapy, which is often simpler and proving effective in chronic diabetic foot ulcers. [14]

Within this backdrop we propose to study the Most Common Organisms Involved In Diabetic Foot Infection And Their Sensitivity To Antimicrobial Agents For The Prevention Of Sepsis/Amputation By The Administration Of Empirical Treatment.

1.1 RATIONALE FOR THE PROJECT

After thoroughly reviewing all the previous research done on the subject

we came to know that the organism responsible for diabetic foot / ulcer is not the same in our setup as in west (Europe/America). [15]

For this reason, we wished to find out the details of this disorder in our setup, including its major causative factors, most common organism and its sensitivity to antimicrobial drugs.

Our research project is directed to meet these objectives.

• Objectives

1. To find out the most common organism responsible for diabetic foot.

- To know their sensitivity to different antimicrobial drugs.
- To find out their resistance to different antimicrobial drugs.
- To find out a sensitive regimen for diabetic foot treatment.
- To establish an empirical treatment based on the findings deduced from these studies.

1.3 Hypothesis

1. Most common organism involved in DF is different in our setup than in West (Europe/America).

2. Resistance/Sensitivity of a drug to an organism depends on the organism isolated.

CHAPTER 2
METHODOLOGY

2.1 STUDY AREA:

Study was carried out to analyze the bacterial isolates of all patients admitted to the:

- **M**edical and **Endocrinology** Ward of **LADY READING HOSPITAL** presented with diabetic foot infection.

- **Surgical** (A, B, C, D, E), **Medical** (A, B, C, D, E) and Orthopedic ward of **KHYBER TEACHING HOSPITAL** presented with diabetic foot infection.

- **Endocrinology** and **Surgical** A ward of **HAYATABAD MEDICAL COMPLEX,** presented with diabetic foot infection.

2.2 STUDY POPULATION:

Population of the study is the people of KPK, visiting these 3 public sector hospitals from different age groups and occupations.

2.3 STUDY DESIGN:

A 2 months long prospective study (taking the midyear population into account) was carried out.

2.4 SAMPLE SIZE:

Sample size is 100

2.5 SAMPLING TECHNIQUE:

Convenient sampling technique is used.

2.6 DATA COLLECTION TECHNIQUE:

A semi structured questionnaire was used for this purpose having open-ended as well as close-ended questions.

In most cases data was collected by person to person interviews with respondents.

2.7 TIME FRAME:

The research was carried out from January 2015 to march 2015.

1

1st week

Topic selection

2

2nd week

Aims & objectives

3

3rdweek

Questionnaire

4

4th-5th week

Data collection

5

6th-7th week

Data analysis & interpretation

6

8th week

Results & finalization

2.8 WORK PLAN:

A simple questionnaire consisting of all related open-ended & close-ended questions was prepared after thorough consultation and approval by project supervisor.

2.9 INCLUSION CRITERIA:

1. Resident of KPK.

2. Admitted in KTH, HMC or LRH for diabetic foot treatment.

2.10 EXCLUSION CRITERIA:

1. Outside KPK's geographical boundaries.

2. Without a confirm diagnosis of diabetes.

2.11 ETHICAL CONSIDERATION:

The questionnaire has been approved by the ethical committee of Khyber Medical College.

2.12 LIMITATIONS OF THE STUDY:

1. Time

2. Finance

3. Resources

4. Lack of co-operation of certain respondents

5. Load shedding

6. Tough routine

7. Use of convenience sampling technique

CHAPTER 3
LITERATURE REVIEW

If you have <u>diabetes</u>, your blood glucose, or <u>blood sugar</u>, levels are too high. Over time, this can damage your nerves or blood vessels. Nerve damage from diabetes can cause you to lose feeling in your feet.

You may not feel a cut, a blister or a sore. Foot injuries such as these can cause ulcers and infections. Serious cases may even lead to amputation.

Damage to the blood vessels can also mean that your feet do not get enough blood and oxygen. It is harder for your foot to heal, if you do get a sore or infection.

You can help avoid foot problems.

First, control your blood sugar levels. Good foot hygiene is also crucial:

- Check your feet every day
- Wash your feet every day
- Keep the skin soft and smooth
- Smooth corns and calluses gently
- If you can see, reach, and feel your feet, trim your toenails regularly. If you cannot, ask a foot doctor (podiatrist) to trim them for you.
- Wear shoes and socks at all times
- Protect your feet from hot and cold
- Keep the blood flowing to your feet

NIH: National Institute of Diabetes and Digestive and Kidney Diseases. [14]

The Diabetic Foot:

If a doctor has ever said you had an elevated blood sugar level even just once when you were pregnant you are at risk for diabetes. About 25 million people have the disease, according to the American Diabetes Association. Nervous system impairment (neuropathy) is a major complication that may cause you to lose feeling in your feet or hands. This means you won't know right away if you hurt yourself. The problem affects about 60 to 70 percent of people with diabetes.

Foot problems are a big risk. All people with diabetes should monitor their feet. If you don't, the consequences can be severe, including amputation. [17]

Diabetic Foot Care Overview:

Diabetes mellitus (DM) represents several diseases in which high blood glucose levels over time can damage the nerves, kidneys, eyes, and blood vessels. Diabetes can also decrease the body's ability to fight infection.

When diabetes is not well controlled, damage to the organs and impairment of the immune system is likely. Foot problems commonly develop in people with diabetes and can quickly become serious.

• With damage to the nervous system, a person with diabetes may not be able to feel his or her feet properly. Normal sweat secretion and oil production that lubricates the skin of the foot is impaired.

• These factors together can lead to abnormal pressure on the skin, bones, and joints of the foot during walking and can lead to breakdown of the skin of the foot. Sores may develop.

• Damage to blood vessels and impairment of the immune system from diabetes makes it difficult to heal these wounds. Bacterial infection of the skin, connective tissues, muscles, and bones can then occur.

• These infections can develop into gangrene. Because of the poor blood flow, antibiotics cannot get to the site of the infection easily. Often, the only treatment for this is amputation of the foot or leg. If the infection spreads to the bloodstream, this process can be life-threatening.

- People with diabetes must be fully aware of how to prevent foot problems before they occur, to recognize problems early, and to seek the right treatment when problems do occur.

- Although treatment for diabetic foot problems has improved, prevention - including good control of blood sugar level - remains the best way to prevent diabetic complications.

People with diabetes should learn how to examine their own feet and how to recognize the early signs and symptoms of diabetic foot problems.

They should also learn what is reasonable to manage routine at home foot care, how to recognize when to call the doctor, and how to recognize when a problem has become serious enough to seek emergency treatment. [18]

Inspection:

- Inspect your feet every day.

- Look for puncture wounds, bruises, pressure areas, redness, warmth, blisters, ulcers, scratches, cuts, and nail problems.

- Get someone to help you, or use a mirror if you are unable to do it alone. You may not feel that damage has occurred to the skin. Inspecting for skin breakdown is crucial.

- Look at and feel each foot for swelling. Swelling in one of the feet and not the other is an early sign that you may be experiencing early stages of Charcot (pronounced "sharko") foot.

- This is a unique problem that can occur in people with nerve damage. It can destroy the bones and joints.

- Examine the bottoms of your feet and toes. Check the six major locations on the bottom of each foot:
  - The tip of the big toe
  - The base of the little toes
  - The base of the middle toes
  - The heel
  - The outside edge of the foot
  - Across the ball of the foot

Shoewear:

Choose and wear your shoes carefully. A poor fitting shoe can cause an ulcer and lead to an infection.

- Buy new shoes late in the day when your feet are larger. Buy shoes that are comfortable without a "breaking in" period.

- Check how your shoe fits in width, length, back, bottom of heel, and sole. Have your feet measured every time you buy new shoes. Your foot will change shape over the years and you may not be the same shoe size you were 5 years ago.

- Avoid pointed-toe styles and high heels. Try to get shoes made with leather upper material and deep toe boxes.

- Wear new shoes for only 2 hours or less at a time. Do not wear the same pair every day.

- Inspect the inside of each shoe before putting it on. Do not lace your shoes too tightly or loosely.

- Avoid long walks without taking a break, removing your shoes and socks and checking for signs of pressure (redness) or ulcers.

Orthotics:

Insurance companies frequently will cover the cost of orthotics for people with diabetes.

They understand how important it is to minimize the risk of a pressure sore in these patients. Discuss this with your primary doctor or orthopedic surgeon.

An accommodative orthotic made from a soft material called plastizote is commonly prescribed. The orthotics should not be hard, as this will increase the risk of a pressure ulcer.

The orthotic can be transferred from shoe to shoe and should be used at all times when standing or walking.

Contributed by: Anish R. Kadakia, MD

Peer-Reviewed by: Stuart J. Fischer, MD; Steven L. Haddad, MD [19]

Motor, sensory and autonomic fibers may all be affected in people with diabetes mellitus.

- Because of sensory deficits, there are no protective symptoms guarding against pressure and heat and so trauma can initiate the development of a leg ulcer.
- Absence of pain contributes to the development of Charcot foot (see below), which further impairs the ability to sustain pressure.
- Motor fiber abnormalities lead to undue physical stress, the development of further anatomical deformities (arched foot, clawing of toes), and contribute to the development of infection.
- When infection complicates a foot ulcer, the combination can be limb-threatening or life-threatening.
- Detection and surveillance of diabetic neuropathy are an essential routine part of a diabetic annual review.

Epidemiology:[20]

- The results of cross-sectional community surveys in the UK showed that 5.3% (type 2) and 7.4% (types 1 and 2 combined) of people with diabetes had a history of active or previous foot ulcer.
- An annual incidence of 2.2% was found in a large community survey in the UK, and up to 7.2% in patients with neuropathy.
- Painful diabetic neuropathy is estimated to affect between 16% and 26% of people with diabetes.[21]
- The incidence of major amputation is between 0.5 and 5.0 per 1,000 people with diabetes.

Risk factors:[22]

• Risk factors for foot ulceration include peripheral arterial disease, peripheral neuropathy, previous amputation, previous ulceration, presence of callus, joint deformity, problems with vision and/or mobility and male sex.Risk factors for peripheral arterial disease include smoking, hypertension and hypercholesterolemia.

Aetiology:

• People with diabetes develop foot ulcers because of neuropathy, ischemia or both.

• The initiating injury may be from acute mechanical or thermal trauma or from repetitively or continuously applied mechanical stress.

• Peripheral neuropathy in people with diabetes results in abnormal forces being applied to the foot, which diabetic ischemia renders the skin less able to withstand.

• Other complications contributing to the onset of ulceration include poor vision, limited joint mobility, and the consequences of cardiovascular and cerebrovascular disease.

• However, the most common precipitant is accidental trauma, especially from ill-fitting footwear.

• Once the skin is broken, many processes contribute to defective healing, including bacterial infection, tissue ischemia, continuing trauma, and poor management.

• Infection can be divided into superficial and local, soft tissue and spreading (cellulitis), and osteomyelitis. Typically, more than one organism is involved, including Gram-positive, Gram-negative, aerobic, and anaerobic species. *Staphylococcus aureus* is the most common pathogen in osteomyelitis.

Charcot foot:

A Charcot foot is a neuro-arthropathic process with osteoporosis, fracture, acute inflammation and disorganization of foot architecture. Suspected Charcot neuro-arthropathy of the foot is an emergency and should be referred immediately to a multidisciplinary foot team [22]

The Charcot foot is characterized by bone and joint degeneration which can lead to a devastating deformity. It usually presents as a hot swollen foot after minor trauma.

Slight trauma triggers fracture of a weakened bone, which increases the load on adjacent bones, leading to gross destruction. The process is self-limiting but the persisting deformity greatly increases the risk of secondary ulceration.

Plain X-ray may be normal but a bone scan may show a hot spot. Damage and developing deformity should be limited by immobilizing the foot in a cast, and realignment arthrodesis of the hind foot can sometimes prevent amputation.

Management: [23]

- Education, including the importance of routine preventative podiatry care, and appropriate footwear. The person should check their feet every day and report any sores or cuts that do not heal, puffiness, swelling, and skin that feel hot to the touch.

- Control of glucose, blood pressure and cholesterol; smoking cessation and weight control.

- Risk assessment.

- Mechanical foot interventions to prevent ulceration.

- Antibiotics to manage and prevent infection.

- Management of peripheral arterial disease, including bypass surgery.

- Wound management, including keeping the wound dry and debridement of dead tissue.

Foot care emergency (new ulceration, swelling, discolouration):

- Don't delay: deterioration in an ulcer is more likely if assessment and management are delayed.

- Take swabs and treat with prompt antibiotics according to local protocols - usually staphylococcal coverage, plus wider spectrum, anaerobes, or streptococcal until sensitivities are known.

- Admit the patient for systemic antibiotic therapy for significant cellulitis or bone infection. Adjust antimicrobial therapy according to culture results when available.

- If osteomyelitis is suspected and initial X-ray does not confirm the presence of osteomyelitis; MRI should be used. If MRI is contra-indicated, white blood cell (WBC) scanning may be performed instead [24]

- If not admitted as an emergency, refer to a multidisciplinary foot care team within 24 hours. A well-organized multidisciplinary approach providing continuity of care between primary and secondary care is essential[25]

Prognosis:

- Foot ulcers in people with diabetes have a high risk of necessitating amputation.

- Ulcer recurrence rates are high, but appropriate education for patients, regular surveillance, the provision of post-healing footwear and regular foot care can reduce rates of re-ulceration.[26]

- Early detection and effective management of diabetic foot ulcers can reduce complications, including preventable amputations and possible mortality.[27]

- Even when healed, diabetic foot should be regarded as a lifelong condition and treated accordingly to prevent recurrence.[28]

- Long-term efforts have reduced amputation rates by 37-75% in different European countries over 10-15 years.[27]

COMPARISON WITH WEST:

"COMMON ORGANISM IN DF BEING DIFFERENT"

Abstract: Metronidazole is the drug of choice for anaerobic infection in diabetic foot ulcers (DFU) for a majority of clinicians. The present study was conducted to determine if Metronidazole is really making a difference in the healing of DFU. *Methods.* Deep tissue samples from the wound area of 61 diabetic foot patients were tested for anaerobic bacterial infection (*Peptostreptococcus productus*, *Bacteroides*, and *Clostridium*) by polymerase chain reaction (PCR). PCR-positive patients were randomized into 2 groups: Metronidazole and non-Metronidazole. Antibiotics for the control of infection were given in both groups as per clinical condition of patients. Treatment outcome was assessed by complete healing of the wound. *Results.* Out of 61 patients, PCR detected evidence of anaerobic infection in 32 (52%), while culture methods detected only 5 (8%) (*Clostridium spp.*), hence emphasizing the significance of the PCR technique over culture methods in detection of microbes. In this study, *Clostridium* was found with maximum prevalence of n (75%), followed by *Bacteroides* with n (53.1%), and *Peptostreptococcus productus* with n (40.6 %). Across all Wagner Ulcer Classification grades, *Clostridium* was the most prevalent anaerobe, and significantly associated with wound age and total leukocyte count. No difference was noted in wound healing in both groups at the end of 16 weeks. *Conclusions.* The authors propose that it is not mandatory to supplement Metronidazole in antibiotic regime for treatment of DFU.[28]

CHAPTER 4
DATA ANALYSIS

This section of analysis revolves around meaningful facts and figures derived computational statistics of our research work.

Our sample size was 100 people belonging to different walks of life with different occupations. 58 were males and 42 were females.

Marital status: 64 were married, 14 were single, 12 were divorced and 10 were widowed.

If we talk about their educational background then 37 were uneducated, 26 studied up to primary, 17 were matriculate and 20 had done higher education.

Demographically, out of the 100 there were 24 from Peshawar region, 5 from DI Khan, 6 each from Chitral and Charsadda, 7 from Nowshera, 8 from Khat, 9 from Bannu, 10 each from Sawabi and Sawat, 15 from FATA.

Occupationally, out of 100 there were 8 who were students, 8 others were self employed, 10 were unemployed, 38 were employed, 36 were house workers.

87 presented with **Type 2 diabetes** and 13 presented with **Type 1 diabetes.**

Amputation: 35 had no amputation, 35 with amputation below ankle, 16 with below knee amputation and 14 with above knee amputation.

HYPOTHESIS 1
ORGANISM:

organisms	Frequency	Percent	Valid Percent	Cumulative Percent
no orgaism	36	36.0	36.0	36.0
E.coli	19	19.0	19.0	55.0
staph aureus	9	9.0	9.0	64.0
MRSA	6	6.0	6.0	70.0
Proteus mirabilis	4	4.0	4.0	74.0

Citrobacter freundii

1

1.0

1.0

75.0

Klebsiella

1

1.0

1.0

76.0

Pseudomonas

7

7.0

7.0

83.0

Acinobacter

2

2.0

2.0

85.0

Coliform species

4

4.0

4.0

89.0

Proteus vulgaris

2

2.0

2.0

91.0

MRSA + E.coli

5

5.0

5.0

96.0

MRSA + pseudomonas

1

1.0

1.0

97.0

staph aureus + coliform species

3

3.0

3.0

100.0

Total

100

100.0

100.0

Pie Chart representing % of organism isolated upon culture

Pie Chart representing FREQUENCY of organism isolated upon culture

HYPOTHESIS 2

BAR CHARTS REPRESENTING SENSITIVITY/ RESISTANCE OF ANTIBIOTICS TO E.COLI:

In the above bar chart piperacillin/ tazobactam being the most sensitive to E. coli strains.

In the above bar chart cefoparazone/ sulbactam being the most sensitive to E. coli strains.

BAR CHARTS REPRESENTING SENSITIVITY/ RESISTANCE OF ANTIBIOTICS TO E.COLI:

In the above bar chart imipenem being the most sensitive to E. coli strains.

BAR CHARTS REPRESENTING SENSITIVITY/ RESISTANCE OF ANTIBIOTICS TO STAPH AUREUS:

In the above bar chart cephtraixone being the most sensitive to E. coli strains.

BAR CHARTS REPRESENTING SENSITIVITY/ RESISTANCE OF ANTIBIOTICS TO STAPH AUREUS:

In the above bar chart tegicyclin being the most sensitive to E. coli strains.

BAR CHARTS REPRESENTING SENSITIVITY/ RESISTANCE OF ANTIBIOTICS TO STAPH AUREUS:

In the above bar chart imipenem, vancomycin and fusidic acid being equally sensitive to Staph aureus strains.

BAR CHARTS REPRESENTING SENSITIVITY/ RESISTANCE OF ANTIBIOTICS TO MRSA:

In the above bar chart MRSA strains resistant to all given antibiotics.

In the above bar chart chloramphenicol, doxycyclin and minocyclin being equally sensitive to MRSA strains.

BAR CHARTS REPRESENTING SENSITIVITY/ RESISTANCE OF ANTIBIOTICS TO MRSA:

In the above bar chart vancomycin being the most sensitive to MRSA strains.

BAR CHARTS REPRESENTING SENSITIVITY/ RESISTANCE OF ANTIBIOTICS TO PSEUDOMONAS:

In the above bar chart piperacillin/ tazobactam being the most sensitive to pseudomonas strains.

In the above bar chart cefoparazone/ sulbactam being the most sensitive to pseudomonas strains.

BAR CHARTS REPRESENTING SENSITIVITY/ RESISTANCE OF ANTIBIOTICS TO PSEUDOMONAS:

In the above bar chart Imipenem being the most sensitive to pseudomonas strains.

BAR CHARTS REPRESENTING SENSITIVITY/ RESISTANCE OF ANTIBIOTICS TO POLYMICROBIAL STRAINS:

In the above bar chart polymicrobial strains resistant to all given antibiotics.

In the above bar chart chloramphenicol being the most sensitive to polymicrobial strains.

BAR CHARTS REPRESENTING SENSITIVITY/ RESISTANCE OF ANTIBIOTICS TO POLYMICROBIAL STRAINS:

In the above bar chart vancomycin being the most sensitive to polymicrobial strains.

PIE CHART SHOWING THE PORTION OF GRAM(+) AND GRAM(-) ORGANISM AMONG THE ONES ISOLATED:

67% were gram negative and 33% were gram positive

Drugs

Organism

E.coli

staph aureus

MRSA

Proteus mirabilis

Citrobacter freundii

Klebsiella

Pseudomonas

Acinobacter

Coliform species

Proteus vulgaris

MRSA + E.coli

MRSA + pseudomonas

staph aureus + coliform species

Total

piperacillin_tazobactam

Resistant

2

0

6

0

1

0

0

2

1

0

5

1

2

20

Sensitive

17

7

0

	4
	0
	1
	7
	0
	3
	2
	0
	0
	0
	41

Total

	19
	7
	6
	4
	1
	1
	7
	2
	4
	2
	5
	1
	2
	61

Percentage

Resistant

	10.5%
	0%
	100%
	0%
	100%
	0%

0%

100%

25%

0%

100%

100%

100%

32.8%

Sensitive

89.5%

100%

0%

100%

0%

100%

100%

0%

75%

100%

0%

O%

0%

67.2%

Amoxicillin

Resistant

9

3

5

2

1

0

1

2

1

2

	4
	2
	32

Sensitive

	4
	4
	0
	1
	0
	1
	2
	0
	2
	0
	0
	1
	15

Total

	13
	7
	5
	3
	1
	1
	3
	2
	3
	2
	4
	3
	47

Percentage

Resistant

	69.2%
	42.8%
	100%
	66.6%
	100%
	0%
	33%
	100%
	33%
	100%
	100%
	66%
	68%

Sensitive

	30.7%
	57.2%
	0%
	33.33%
	0%
	1005
	66%
	0%
	66%
	0%
	0%
	33%
	32%

Augmentin

Resistant

	16
	2

6

1

1

1

6

2

2

1

5

1

2

46

Sensitive

0

7

0

3

0

0

1

0

2

1

0

0

1

15

Total

16

9

6

4

1

1

		7
		2
		4
		2
		5
		1
		3
		61

Percentage

Resistant

		100%
		22.2%
		100%
		25%
		100%
		100%
		85.8%
		100%
		50%
		50%
		100%
		100%
		66%
		75.4%

Sensitive

		0%
		77.8%
		0%
		75%
		0%
		0%
		14.2%
		0%
		50%
		50%

0%

0%

33%

24.6%

Cepherdine

Resistant

13

0

6

2

1

1

4

2

4

2

4

1

2

42

Sensitive

6

8

0

2

0

0

3

0

0

0

0

0

1

20

Total

19

8

6

4

1

1

7

2

4

2

4

1

3

62

Percentage

Resistant

68.4%

0%

100%

50%

100%

100%

57.1%

100%

100%

100%

4%

100%

66%

67.8%

Sensitive

31.65

100%

0%

50%

0%

0%

42.9%

0%

0%

0%

0%

0%

33%

32.2%

Cefuroxime

resistance

12

0

3

2

1

1

4

2

4

2

3

2

36

Sensitive

6

7

0

2

0

0

3

0

0

0

0

0

18

Total

18

7

3

4

1

1

7

2

4

2

3

2

54

Percentage
Resistant

66%

0%

100%

50%

100%

100%

57.1%

100%

100%

100%

100%

100%

66%

Sensitive

33%

100%

0%

50%

0%

0%

42,9%

0%

0%

0%

0%

0%

33%

Cephtriaxone

Resistance

11

0

5

0

1

1

4

2

2

2

5

1

2

36

Sensitive

7
9
0
4
0
0
3
0
2
0
0
0
1
26

Total

18
9
5
4
1
1
7
2
4
2
5
1
3
62

Percentage
Resistant

61.1%
0%

100%

0%

100%

100%

57.1%

100%

50%

100%

100%

100%

66%

58%

Sensitive

38.9%

100%

0%

100%

0%

0%

42.9%

0%

50%

0%

0%

0%

33%

42%

Cefutoxime

Resistance

13

0

6

0

1

1

4

2

2

2

3

1

2

37

Sensitive

5

9

0

4

0

0

3

0

2

0

0

0

1

24

Total

18

9

6

4

1

1

7

2

4

2

	3
	1
	3
	61

Percentage

Resistant

	72.2%
	0%
	100%
	0%
	100%
	100%
	57.1%
	100%
	50%
	100%
	100%
	100%
	66%
	60.6%

Sensitive

	27.8%
	100%
	0%
	100%
	0%
	0%
	42.9%
	0%
	50%
	0%
	0%
	0%
	33%
	39.4%

Cefpodoxime

Resistance

	12
	0
	3
	0
	1
	1
	3
	2
	2
	2
	3
	2
	31

Sensitive

	7
	8
	0
	4
	0
	0
	4
	0
	1
	0
	0
	0
	24

Total

	19
	8

3

4

1

1

7

2

3

2

3

2

55

Percentage

Resistant

63.1%

0%

100%

O%

100%

100%

42.9%

100%

66%

100%

100%

100%

56.4%

Sensitive

36.9%

100%

0%

100%

0%

0%

57.1%

0%

33%

0%

0%

0%

43.6%

Ceftazidime

Resistane

12

0

3

0

1

0

3

2

2

2

3

2

30

Sensitive

7

7

0

4

0

1

4

0

2

0

Total

0

0

25

19

7

3

4

1

1

7

2

4

2

3

2

55

Percentage
Resistant

63.1%

0%

100%

0%

100%

0%

42.9%

100%

50%

100%

100%

100%

54.6%

Sensitive

36.9%

100%

0%

100%

0%

100%

57.1%

0%

50%

0%

0%

0%

45.4%

Cefepime

Resistane

10

0

3

0

1

1

3

2

2

2

3

2

29

Sensitive

7

7

0

4

0

0

4

0

1

0

0

0

23

Total

17

7

3

4

1

1

7

2

3

2

3

2

52

Percentage
Resistant

58.8%

0%

100%

0%

100%

100%

42.9%

100%

66%

100%

100%

100%

55.8%

Sensitive

41.2%

100%

0%

100%

0%

0%

57.1%

0%

33%

0%

0%

44.2%

Cefoperazone/ sulbactam

Resistant

1

0

2

0

1

1

3

1

2

0

3

2

16

Sensitive

17

7

0

4

0

0

4

1

2

2

0

0

37

Total

18

7

2

4

1

1

7

2

4

2

3

2

53

Percentage

Resistant

	5.6%
	0%
	100%
	0%
	100%
	100%
	42.9%
	50%
	50%
	0%
	100%
	100%
30.2%	

Sensitive

	94.4%
	100%
	0%
	100%
	0%
	0%
	57.1%
	50%
	50%
	100%
	0%
	0%
	69.8%

Polymixin-B

Resistane

	3
	0

	1
	0
	0
	0
	2
	1
	2
	1
	3
	2
	15
Sensitive	
	10
	7
	0
	3
	1
	1
	4
	1
	2
	0
	0
	0
	29
Total	
	13
	7
	1
	3
	1
	1

6

2

4

1

3

2

44

Percentage

Resistant

23.1%

0%

100%

0%

0%

0%

33%

50%

50%

100%

100%

100%

34%

Sensitive

76.9%

100%

0%

100%

100%

100%

66%

50%

50%

0%

	Colestin Resistane	Sensitive
	0%	
	0%	
	66%	
	2	11
	0	7
	1	0
	0	3
	0	1
	0	1
	1	4
	1	1
	1	2
	3	0
	2	0
	11	30

	Total

Total

13
7
1
3
1
1
5
2
3

3

2
41

Percentage
Resistant

15.4%
0%
100%
0%
0%
0%
20%
50%
33%

100%

100%
26.8%

Sensitive

84.6%
100%

	0%
	100%
	100%
	100%
	80%
	50%
	66%
	0%
	0%
	73.2%

Cotrimoxazole

Resistane

	9
	4
	2
	3
	1
	1
	2
	2
	2
	5
	1
	2
	34

Sensitive

	4
	4
	3
	1
	0
	0

3

0

1

0

0

1

17

Total

13

8

5

4

1

1

5

2

3

5

1

3

51

Percentage
Resistant

69.2%

50%

40%

75%

100%

100%

40%

100%

66%

100%

100%

66%

66.7%

Sensitive

30.7%

50%

60%

25%

0%

0%

60%

0%

33%

0%

0%

33%

33.3%

Chloramphenicol

Resistane

5

1

0

0

1

0

2

2

2

1

0

1

15

Sensitive

8

8

6

3

0

1

3

0

2

4

1

2

38

Total

13

9

6

3

1

1

5

2

4

5

1

3

53

Percentage
Resistant

38.4%

11.1%

0%

0%

100%

0%

40%

100%

50%

20%

0%

33%

28.3%

Sensitive

61.5%

88.9%

100%

100%

0%

100%

60%

0%

50%

80%

100%

66%

71.7%

Doxycycline

Resistane

5

2

0

1

1

0

1

2

3

2

0

1

18

Sensitive

7

6

6

2

0

1

4

0

0

2

1

2

31

Total

12

8

6

3

1

1

5

2

3

4

1

3

49

Percentage

Resistant

41.7%

25%

0%

33%

100%

0%

20%

100%

100%

50%

0%

33%

36.7%

Sensitive

58.3%

75%

100%

66%

0%

100%

80%

0%

0%

50%

100%

66%

63.3%

Minocycline

Resistane

4

2

0

1

1

0

1

2

2

2

0

1

16

Sensitive

7

6

6

2

0

1

4

0

0

2

1

2

31

total

11

8

	6
	3
	1
	1
	5
	2
	2
	4
	1
	3
	47

Percentage

Resistant

	36.4%
	25%
	0%
	33%
	100%
	0%
	20%
	100%
	100%
	50%
	0%
	33%
	34%

.

Sensitive

	63.6%
	75%
	100%
	66%
	0%
	100%

80%

0%

0%

50%

100%

66%

66%

Ciprofloxacin

Resistane

13

3

2

0

1

0

4

2

2

0

4

1

3

35

Sensitive

5

6

0

3

0

1

3

0

2

2

0

0

0

22

Total

18

9

2

3

1

1

7

2

4

2

4

1

3

57

Percentage

Resistant

72.2%

33%

100%

0%

100%

0%

57.1%

100%

50%

0%

100%

100%

100%

61.4%

Sensitive

27.8%

66%

0%

100%

0%

100%

42.9%

0%

50%

100%

0%

0%

0%

38.6%

Levofloxacin

Resistane

9

1

2

0

1

0

4

2

2

0

4

1

3

29

Sensitive

9

7

	0
	4
	0
	1
	3
	0
	2
	1
	0
	0
	0
Total	27

	18
	8
	2
	4
	1
	1
	7
	2
	4
	1
	4
	1
	3
	56

Percentage
Resistant

	50%
	12.5%
	100%
	0%
	100%
	0%

57.1%

100%

50%

0%

100%

100%

100%

51.8%

Sensitive

50%

87.5%

0%

100%

0%

100%

42.9%

0%

50%

100%

0%

0%

0%

48.2%

Tegicyclin

Resistane

1

0

1

0

1

0

1

2

0

0

3

2

11

Sensitive

15

8

3

3

0

1

3

0

2

2

2

1

40

Total

16

8

4

3

1

1

4

2

2

2

5

3

51

Percentage

Resistant

	6.3%
	0%
	25%
	0%
	100%
	0%
	25%
	100%
	0%
	0%
	60%
	66%
	21.6%

Sensitive

	93.7%
	100%
	75%
	100%
	0%
	100%
	75%
	0%
	100%
	100%
	40%
	33%
	78.4%

Amikacin

Resistant

	2
	2

	0
	0
	1
	0
	3
	1
	2
	1
	2
	0
	14

Sensitive

	16
	5
	1
	4
	0
	1
	4
	1
	2
	0
	2
	2
	38

Total

	18
	7
	1
	4
	1
	1

	7
	2
	4
	1
	4
	2
	52

Percentage

Resistant

	11.1%
	71.4%
	0%
	0%
	100%
	0%
	42.9%
	50%
	50%
	100%
	50%
	0%
	26.9%

Sensitive

	88.9%
	28.6%
	100%
	100%
	0%
	100%
	57.1%
	50%
	50%
	0%

50%

100%

73.1%

Imipenem

Resistant

2

0

5

0

1

0

2

2

1

0

5

2

20

Sensitive

17

7

0

3

0

1

5

0

3

2

0

0

38

	Total	Percentage Resistant	Sensitive
	19	10.5%	89.5%
	7	0%	100%
	5	100%	
	3	0%	
	1	100%	
	1	0%	
	7	28.6%	
	2	100%	
	4	25%	
	2	0%	
	5	100%	
	2	100%	
	58	34.5%	

0%

100%

0%

100%

71.4%

0%

75%

100%

0%

0%

65.5%

Vancomycin

Resistant

1

0

0

0

1

0

1

1

0

0

0

0

1

5

Sensitive

12

7

6

3

0

1

	3
	1
	1
	1
	5
	1
	1
	42

Total

	13
	7
	6
	3
	1
	1
	4
	2
	1
	1
	5
	1
	2
	47

Percentage

Resistant

	7.7%
	0%
	0%
	0%
	100%
	0%
	25%
	50%
	0%
	0%

	0%
	0%
	50%
	10.6%

Sensitive

	92.3%
	100%
	100%
	100%
	0%
	100%
	75%
	50%
	100%
	100%
	100%
	100%
	50%
	89.4%

Fusidic acid

Resistant

	1
	1
	0
	0
	1
	0
	1
	1
	0
	0
	1
	0
	2
	8

Sensitive

12
7
4
3
0
1
3
1
1
1
4
1
1
39

Total

13
8
4
3
1
1
4
2
1
1
5
1
3
47

Percentage
Resistant

7.7%
12.5%

0%

0%

100%

0%

25%

50%

0%

0%

20%

0%

66%

17%

Sensitive

92.3%

87.5%

100%

100%

0%

100%

75%

50%

100%

100%

80%

100%

33%

83%

OBJECTIVE 1:

To find out the most common organism responsible for diabetic foot.

The three most frequently found **Aerobic** bacteria *E.coli (19%), Staph. Aureus (9%), Psedomonas (7%)*

The most frequently found **Gram positive** bacteriae are *Staph. Aureus (9%), MRSA (6%)*

The most common **Gram negative bacteriae** are *E.coli (19%), Psedomonas (7%), Proteus (4%)*

OBJECTIVE 2:

To know their sensitivity to different antimicrobial drugs.

Gram **positive**; **Cefelosporins {Generation ll and lll (100%) }, Vancomycin(100%), Imipinem(100%), Pipracilline/Tazobectam (100%)**

Gram **negative**; **Cefoperazone/Tazobactam (94.4%), Vancomycin (92.3%), Imipenem (89.4%), Piperacilline/Tazobectam (89.4%)**

MRSA ;Vancomycin(100%), Chloramphenicol(100%), Amikacin(100%), Minocyclin(100%)

polymicrobial infection; **Vancomycin (100%), Chloramphenicol (80%), amikacin (50%)**

OBJECTIVE 3:

To find out their resistance to different antimicrobial drugs.

The most resistant drugs to the majority of isolated organisms:

- Augmentin
- Ciprofloxacin
- Levofloxacin
- Cephradine
- cotrimoxazole

OBJECTIVE 4:

To find out a sensitive regimen for diabetic foot treatment

Most effective drugs against Gram **positive** are *Cefelosporins {Generation ll and lll (100%) }, Vancomycin(100%), Imipinem(100%), Pipracilline/Tazobectam (100%)*

Most effective drugs against Gram **negative** are *Cefoperazone/Tazobactam (94.4%), Vancomycin (92.3%), Imipenem (89.4%), Piperacilline/Tazobectam (89.4%)*

Most effective drugs against **MRSA** are *Vancomycin(100%), Chloramphenicol(100%), Amikacin(100%), Minocyclin(100%)*

Most effective drug against **polymicrobial infection** are *Vancomycin (100%), Chloramphenicol (80%), amikacin (50%)*

OBJECTIVE 5:

To establish an empirical treatment based on the findings deduced from these studies.

We suggest an empirical treatment based on:

- Amikacin
- Vancomycin

- Piperacillin/ tazobactam
- Chloramphenicol
- Imipenem

DEMOGRAPHICAL DISTRIBUTION:

Demographically, out of the 100 there were 24 from Peshawar region, 5 from DI Khan, 6 each from Chitral and Charsadda, 7 from Nowshera, 8 from Khat, 9 from Bannu, 10 each from Sawabi and Sawat, 15 from FATA.

OCCUPATION:

Out of 100 there were 8 who were students, 8 others were self employed, 10 were unemployed, 38 were employed, 36 were house workers.

AGE WISE DISTRIBUTION:

ORGANISM DISTRIBUTION VS REGION:

TYPE OF DIABETES:

87 presented with **Type 2 diabetes** and 13 presented with **Type 1 diabetes.**

AMPUTATION:

35 had no amputation, 35 with amputation below ankle, 16 with below knee amputation and 14 with above knee amputation.

EDUCATIONAL STATUS: If we talk about their educational background then 37 were uneducated, 26 studied up to primary, 17 were matriculate and 20 had done higher education.

Marital status:

64 were married, 14 were single, 12 were divorced and 10 were widowed.

GENDER AFFECTED:

Our sample size was 100 people belonging to different walks of life with different occupations. 58 were males and 42 were females.

CHAPTER 5
DISCUSSION

This study is done to assess the **organisms** involve in diabetic foot infection and their **sensitivity** to antimicrobial agents.

Bacteriological specimens were obtained and processed using standard hospital procedure for microbiological culture and sensitivity testing.

Cultures grown in aerobic incubation at 37 degree Celsius.

RESULTS:

A **total** of 100 {62 **aerobes** (62%) and 38 **others** (fungal or **anaerobes**) (38%)} were isolated.

Gram positive 47 (75.8%) and Gram negative 15(24.2%)

Polymicrobial infections 9(9%)

The three most frequently found **Aerobic** bacteria *E.coli (19%), Staph. Aureus (9%), Pseudomonas (7%)*

The most frequently found **Gram positive** bacteria are *Staph. Aureus (9%), MRSA (6%)*

The most common **Gram negative bacteria** are *E.coli (19%), Pseudomonas (7%), and Proteus (4%)*

Most effective drugs against Gram **positive** are *Cephalosporin's {Generation ll and lll (100%)}, Vancomycin (100%), Imipenem (100%), Piperacilline/Tazobectam (100%)*

Most effective drugs against Gram **negative** are *Cefoperazone/Sulbactam (94.4%), Vancomycin (92.3%), Imipenem (89.4%), and Piperacilline/Tazobectam (89.4%)*

Most effective drugs against **MRSA** are *Vancomycin (100%), Chloramphenicol (100%), Amikacin (100%), and Minocyclin (100%)*

Most effective drug against **polymicrobial infection** is *Vancomycin (100%), Chloramphenicol (80%), and amikacin (50%).*

CHAPTER 5
CONCLUSION

Staph. Aureus and **E.coli** are the most common Gram positive and Gram negative organisms, respectively, in KPK.

Anaerobes are still the most common cause for this infection, although the prevalence is less.

These ulcers and infections may require use of combined antimicrobial therapy for initial management, repeated dressing and wound debridement may be required.

This study helps us to choose empirical treatment for patients with diabetic foot infection and also in the management of patient who comes with sepsis that is caused from diabetic foot.

CHAPTER 5
RECOMMENDATIONS

From our study, we can concoct the following recommendations which show us the most common organism involved in the diabetic foot and help us in preventing the amputation and sepsis.

- Since the most common organism appears to be E.coli and it is most sensitive to drugs such as;

  - *Cefoperazone/Sulbactam (94.4%)*

  - *Vancomycin (92.3%)*

  - *Imipenem (89.4%)*

  - *Piperacilline/Tazobectam (89.4%)*

- **Therefore, patients presenting with diabetic foot should be directly put on empirical treatment, to prevent further damage to the body and better recovery.**

- **The patients should be educated to keep their feet clean and healthy.**

- **The attendants of the patients should be advised to take proper care of their patient.**

- **The patient should be compelled to check their limbs specially lower extremities for any ulcers, wounds or cuts.**

- Good compliance to therapy will yield positive results and would eradicate the complications before it causes further damage to health.

CHAPTER 5
REFERENCES

- Detection of Anaerobic Infection in Diabetic Foot Ulcer Using PCR Technique and the Status of Metronidazole Therapy on Treatment Outcome.

http://www.woundsresearch.com/article/detection-anaerobic-infection-diabetic-foot-ulcer-using-pcr-technique-and-status-metronidazo

Issue: Volume 24 - Issue 10 - October 2012

Index: WOUNDS. 2012;24(10):283–288.

- Boulton in Diabetes, 30;36 2002

- Lipsky BA. Evidence-based antibiotic therapy of diabetic foot infections. *FEMS Immunol Medical Microbiol.* 1999;26:267-276.

- Deresinski S. Infections in the diabetic patient: Strategies for the clinician. *Infectious Disease Reports*. 1995;1(1): 1-12.

- Issue: Volume 24 - Issue 10 - October 2012

Index: WOUNDS. 2012;24(10):283–288.

- Singh, N. "Preventing Foot Ulcers in Patients With Diabetes". JAMA. Retrieved 21 November 2013.

- Arad Y, Fonseca V, Peters A, Vinik A (2011). "Beyond the Monofilament for the Insensate Diabetic Foot: A systematic review of randomized trials to prevent the occurrence of plantar foot ulcers in patients with diabetes". *Diabetes Care* 34 (4): 1041–6. doi:10.2337/dc10-1666. PMC 3064020. PMID 21447666. http://en.wikipedia.org/wiki/Diabetic_foot#cite_note-pmid21447666-5

- "Antibiotics Guide". Retrieved August 16, 2014. http://en.wikipedia.org/wiki/Diabetic_foot#cite_note-6

- Brem, H.; Tomic-Canic, M. (2007). "Cellular and molecular basis of wound healing in diabetes". *Journal of Clinical Investigation* 117 (5): 1219–1222. doi:10.1172/JCI32169.PMC 1857239. PMID 17476353

- Iakovos N Nomikos et al, Protective and Damaging Aspects of Healing: A Review,*Wounds* 2006; 18 (7) 177-185.

- McLennan S et al, Molecular aspects of wound healing, Primary intention(2006).14(1) 8-13. http://en.wikipedia.org/wiki/Diabetic_foot_ulcer#cite_note-Iakovos-2

- Blume, P. A.; Walters, J.; Payne, W.; Ayala, J.; Lantis, J. (2008). "Comparison of Negative Pressure Wound Therapy Using Vacuum-Assisted Closure with Advanced Moist Wound Therapy in the Treatment of Diabetic Foot Ulcers: A multicenter randomized controlled trial". *Diabetes Care* 31 (4): 631–636. doi:10.2337/dc07-2196.PMID 18162494

- Sharman Debbie (2003). "Moist wound healing: a review of evidence, application and outcome". *The Diabetic Foot* 6 (3): 112–120.

- Jørgensen, Bo; Tonny Karlsmark, Hanne Vogensen, Lone Haase and Rasmus Lundquist (18 October 2011). "A Pilot Study of Leucopatch, an Autologous, Additive-Free, Platelet-Rich Fibrin for the Treatment of Recalcitrant Chronic Wounds to Determine Safety". *The International Journal of Lower Extremity Wounds.*

- http://www.woundsresearch.com/article/detection-anaerobic-infection-diabetic-foot-ulcer-using-pcr-technique-and-status-metronidazo

- http://www.nlm.nih.gov/medlineplus/diabeticfoot.html

- http://www.aofas.org/footcaremd/conditions/diabetic-foot/Pages/default.aspx

- *Medically Reviewed by a Doctor on 5/29/2014*

Medical Author: Robert Ferry Jr., MD Medical Editor: Melissa Conrad Stöppler, MD, Chief Medical Editor

http://www.emedicinehealth.com/diabetic_foot_care/article_em.htm

- Last reviewed: December 2011*Contributed by: Anish R. Kadakia, MD Peer-Reviewed by: Stuart J. Fischer, MD; Steven L. Haddad, MD http://orthoinfo.aaos.org/topic.cfm?topic=A00148*

- Jeffcoate WJ, Harding KG; Diabetic foot ulcers. Lancet. 2003 May 3;361(9368):1545-51.

- Neuropathic pain – pharmacological management: The pharmacological management of neuropathic pain in adults in non-specialist settings; NICE Clinical Guideline (Nov 2013)

- Management of diabetes; Scottish Intercollegiate Guidelines Network - SIGN (March 2010)

- Type 2 diabetes: Prevention and management of foot problems; NICE Clinical Guideline (January 2004)

- Diabetes - type 2; NICE CKS, July 2010 (UK access only)

- Diabetic foot problems - inpatient management; NICE Clinical Guideline (March 2011)

- Cavanagh PR, Lipsky BA, Bradbury AW, et al; Treatment for diabetic foot ulcers. Lancet. 2005 Nov 12;366(9498):1725-35.

- Lewis J, Lipp A; Pressure-relieving interventions for treating diabetic foot ulcers. Cochrane Database Syst Rev. 2013 Jan 31;1:CD002302. doi: 10.1002/14651858.CD002302.pub2.

- Detection of Anaerobic Infection in Diabetic Foot Ulcer Using PCR Technique and the Status of Metronidazole Therapy on Treatment Outcome.
http://www.woundsresearch.com/article/detection-anaerobic-infection-diabetic-foot-ulcer-using-pcr-technique-and-status-metronidazo

Issue: Volume 24 - Issue 10 - October 2012

Index: WOUNDS. 2012;24(10):283–288.

ANNEXURE

To Find The Most Common Organisms Involved In Diabetic Foot Infection And Their

Sensitivity To Antimicrobial Agents For The Prevention Of Sepsis/Amputation By The Administration Of Empirical Treatment.

QUESTIONAIRE

BIODATA

NAME _____   SEX _____

AGE _____

ADDRESS _____   OCCUPATION

_____

MARRIED/UNMARRIED _____   EDUCATION

_____

DIABETES MELLITIS HISTORY

DURATION _____

MEAN RBS _____

ANY COMPLICATIONS _____

DIABETIC FOOT HISTORY

GRADE _____

ANY AMPUTATION (Tick one option)

1. Below ankle

 2. Below knee

3. Above knee

CULTURE AND SENSITIVITY REPORT

ORGANISIM INVOLVE _____

SENSITIVE TO

Amoxicilline   Polymixin B

Co-amoxiclave   Amikacin

Piperacilline/Tazobactam   Cotrimaxazole

Cephradine   Chloramphenicol

Cefuroxime   Tegicyclin

Cephtriaxone   Ticarcilin/Clavulanic
Acid

Cefotaxime   Ciprofloxacin

Cefodoxime   Sparfloxacin

Ceftazidime   Levofloxacin

Cefipim	Meropenem
Cefoparazone/Sulbactam	Imipenem
Fusidic Acid	Vancomycin

KEY

S= Sensitivity

R = Resistant

PERMISSION LETTER FOR DATA COLLECTION

DEPARTMENT OF COMMUNITY MEDICINE KHYBER MEDICAL COLLEGE PESHAWAR

Ph: 9216206-09

Ext: 168

Date._____/_____/ 2015

TO

SUBJECT: **_FACILITATION FOR THE COLLECTION OF DATA._**

It is respectfully stated that the 4th year MBBS students of Khyber Medical College(batch #__) have been allotted a research project "
__".

They are advised to collect data about _____.

It is requested that you kindly allow them to collect the required data. Your help in this regard will be highly appreciated.

Thanking You.

Dr. Bushra iftikhar

Professor/ Head

Dept. of Community Medicine

Khyber Medical College, Peshawar.